Indwelling Catheter

I0469051

By Sharon C Kelly, Registered Nurse

Are you caring for someone at home who has an indwelling urinary catheter? Do you have concerns about how to take care of a person with a catheter? This article will give you all the information you need to be comfortable in the care of that person. There are a number of reasons why someone would need a need a urinary catheter at home. Catheters are used to drain the bladder of someone who cannot do that naturally.

How many of us take our urinary systems for granted? When we feel the need to pee, we go empty our bladder. If a person is unable to empty their bladder, or is unable to control the leakage of urine and therefore has rashes and sores because their skin has constant contact with urine, a long term indwelling catheter might be the answer. Another reason someone might have a catheter is because of a medical condition such as multiple sclerosis or a spinal cord injury. With these diseases a bladder can become nonfunctional. Also, a catheter may be placed in someone with a terminal illness as a matter of comfort.

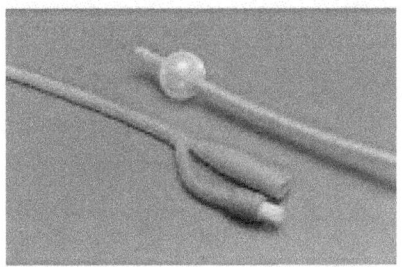

A long term urinary catheter is placed in someone only when it is absolutely necessary because of the risks involved. The biggest risk is the introduction of pathogens (germs) into the bladder. Bacterial growth is common at the catheter insertion site. Once an infection occurs in the bladder, it can then travel up into the kidneys. Other risks include; injury to the urethra, blockage of the catheter, skin breakdown at the tip of the penis, accidental catheter dislodgement with balloon inflated. I will be discussing these risks and what can be done to avoid them a little further along in this article.

Glossary of terms

Catheter Associated Urinary Tract Infection: (CAUTI): This type of infection is caused by pathogens that get into the body along the catheter tube or get into the body by getting inside the catheter tube. This can happen when the closed drainage system is opened.

Closed drainage system: Once the indwelling catheter is in place, and the tubing is connected to the drainage bag, the tubing should never be disconnected.

Fluid Intake: All patients with catheters should have a daily intake of 2000-2500 ml. if permitted by Doctor.

Incontinence: The inability to control bladder or bowels.

Indwelling or Foley catheter: A drainage tube that is anchored in place in the bladder by a balloon.

Meatus: A body opening or passage, such as the opening of the urethral canal.

Microorganism: A living thing that is so small it cannot be seen with the naked eye.

Suprapubic catheterization: A surgical placement of a catheter through the abdominal wall into the urinary bladder. Urine drains into a drainage bag.

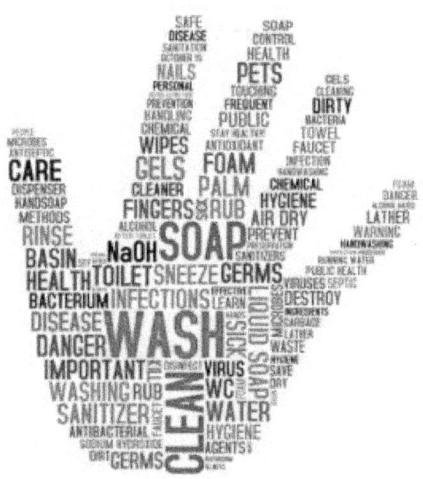

Handwashing

Proper handwashing is the number one way to prevent infections!

Always wash your hands before and after handling the catheter. It is important to wash your hands properly in order to protect yourself and the person you are caring for from infection.

The following steps are taken directly from the Centers for Disease Control (CDC) website:

The right way to wash your hands!

- Wet your hands with clean, running water (warm or cold) and apply soap.
- Rub your hands together to make lather and scrub them well; be sure to scrub the backs of your hands, between your fingers, and under your nails.
- Continue rubbing your hands for at least 20 seconds. Need a timer? Hum the "Happy Birthday" song from beginning to end twice.
- Rinse your hands well under running water.
- Dry your hands using a clean towel or air dry them.

Washing hands with soap and water is the best way to reduce the number of germs on them. If soap and water are not available, use an alcohol-based sanitizer that contains at least 60% alcohol. Alcohol-based hand sanitizers can quickly reduce the number of germs on hands in some situations, but they do **not** eliminate all types of germs.

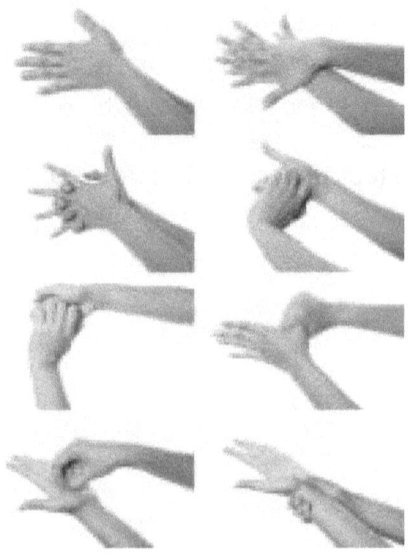

Catheter Care

Catheter care needs to be performed every day. It should also be performed after every bowel movement or any time there are secretions present at the catheter insertion site.

Gather supplies: Washcloth, towel, soap and warm water or other cleaning solution, disposable gloves

Procedure: Wash hands and put on disposable gloves. If perineal (genital area) care has not already been done, it can be done along with catheter care. Before giving any care, observe the catheter area for any crusting, lesions, discharge or anything abnormal. This is an essential part of the catheter care. Also, do not use powders or lotions on the genital area because there is a risk of infection.

For a female patient:

- Gently separate the labia and wash the entire area around where the catheter enters the meatus. Always wash from the cleanest part to the dirtiest part. If also doing perineal care, always wash from front to back.
- With one hand, hold the catheter steady near the meatus (don't push it farther up the urethra.) If it gets pushed up, germs can be introduced into the urinary tract. With the other hand wash down the catheter about 4" from the meatus. Never wash the catheter upward toward the meatus. This is bringing dirty into clean.
- Rinse and dry the catheter the same way as you washed it.

For a male patient:

- Gently pull back the foreskin, if the patient is uncircumcised, and wash the entire area. Use a circular motion when washing the meatus and glans. Gently replace the foreskin if you have pulled it back.
- Hold the catheter near the meatus with on hand while you use the other hand to wash down the catheter for about 4" from the meatus. Do not push the catheter farther up in the urethra. This increases the risk of germs getting in to the urinary tract. Never wash up the catheter toward the meatus.
- Rinse and dry the catheter the same way as you washed it.

You may shower while wearing a catheter, but **do not** take a tub bath.

For someone with a catheter, it is important to make sure the drainage bag is always below the level of the person's bladder. Urine must never flow from the bag or tubing back into the bladder. This can cause an infection. Also, check the tubing for kinks and twists or the person lying or sitting on the tubing. This can prevent the urine from draining.

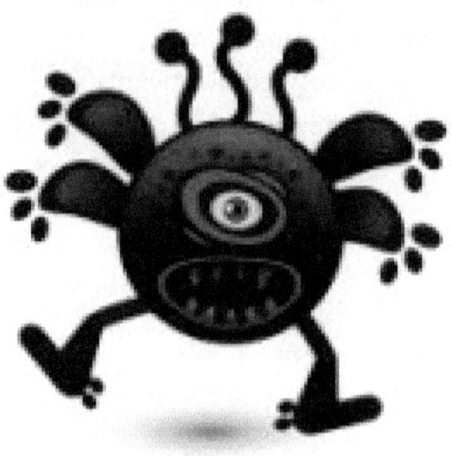

Emptying the Catheter Bag

Always empty the catheter drainage bag when it is ½ to 2/3 full. If it is allowed to get too full, it can pull on and injure the urethra.

Gather supplies: measuring container, paper towels, disposable gloves, alcohol wipes

Procedure for large volume (night) catheter bag:

- Wash your hands.
- Put on gloves.
- Place paper towel on floor under the drainage bag.
- Always keep drainage bag off of the floor.
- Place measuring container on paper towel.
- Open the drain on bag without letting the open end touch anything.
- Hold drain while urine flows out of bag into the measuring container.
- When urine all the urine has drained, close the drain and wipe the end of the drain with an alcohol swab. Replace the drain tube in its holder on the catheter bag.
- Be sure to note the amount appearance and odor of the urine.
- Empty urine in toilet.
- Clean and store the measuring container.
- Remove and dispose of gloves.
- Wash your hands.

Procedure for emptying leg bag:

- Undo bottom strap of leg bag.
- Hold the bottom end of the bag up.
- Open the bag by turning the spout or by removing the cap.
- Drain into container. Note appearance and odor of the urine.
- Replace the cap or screw tight. Strap bag to leg.

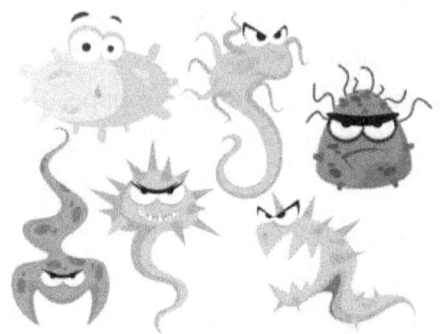

Changing Night bag to leg bag

For a person who is up and around during the day, changing from a bedside drainage bag to a leg bag is an option. The leg bag will need to be emptied more often, but you can move around freely with it and it can be hidden under your pants or skirt. It is important to remember that whatever bag you are using, it must be kept below the level of the bladder. (Hip level)

Gather supplies: leg bag, alcohol pads, disposable gloves, paper towels or clean towel

Procedure:

- Wipe all the connections with an alcohol wipe before disconnecting the tubing.
- Take the cap off of the clean leg bag. Wipe the opening with an alcohol wipe and place bag on clean towel.
- Pinch the catheter tubing (this is the tubing coming out of the meatus) in order to stop the flow of urine while you disconnect the tubing.
- Disconnect the tubing from the catheter being very careful not to let the end of it touch anything.
- Wipe the end of the catheter with alcohol wipe and connect it to the leg bag.
- Secure the catheter tubing to the thigh leaving enough slack so that it doesn't pull on the meatus.
- Secure the leg bag to the calf. Adjust the straps so that they are comfortable and not too tight.
- Empty large drainage bag and clean and store until bedtime. It must be cleaned whenever removed to help prevent infection and eliminate odor.

Cleaning Drainage Bags

Drainage bags need to be cleaned daily. This is if you are changing bags from day to night or night to day.

Gather supplies: household bleach solution (2 tablespoons to 1 quart water) or vinegar solution (2 parts white vinegar to 3 parts water), catheter tipped syringe, disposable gloves, and towel

Procedure: Mix your solution first (use new solution each time)

- Wash your hands.
- Rinse bag thoroughly with hot water and empty. Always put solution through top and empty from bottom.
- Fill bag about 2/3 full with cleaning solution and soak for about 30 minutes.
- After soaking, empty the bag.
- Using the catheter syringe inject enough air into the bag, so that the sides of the bag are not sticking together. This will allow adequate drying.
- Store on clean towel.

Positioning Urinary Drainage Bags

 The most important thing to remember about positioning a catheter drainage bag is to always keep it below the level of the bladder. I know I have said this before, but it is so very important that it bears repeating.

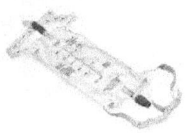

Leg Bags

- Always apply leg bags to the calf.
- Alternate legs each day.
- Always apply the leg bag with the anti - reflux valve at the top. This valve prevents the urine from going back into the bladder from the leg bag.
- Make sure the leg bag – connecting tubing is short enough to prevent kinking, and long enough to prevent pulling on the catheter

Bedside Drainage Bag (large volume bag)

- Keep the tubing coiled on the bed. Do not let the tubing hang below the drainage bag.
- Connect the drainage bag to the bed frame. (not a movable part of the bed) Do not allow the bag to lie on the floor.

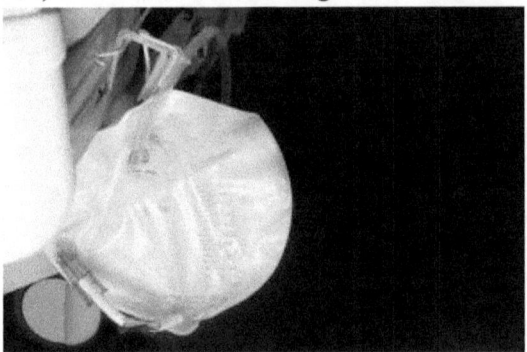

Flushing the Catheter or Not

In order to keep the urine flowing freely from the bladder into the drainage bag, it is sometimes necessary to flush the catheter with a sterile solution. This could be necessary if the catheter becomes plugged with pus or sediment. Also, if you notice that your output is much less than your intake and you have checked the position of tubing and bag and everything looks to be okay. However, if these things do happen, it is best to have the catheter changed rather than flush it because flushing the catheter washes the pus and sediment back into the bladder and can create a worse infection. If urine is not draining freely, try milking the tubing. This is done by squeezing and then releasing the tubing, starting at a point close to the patient and going outward toward the drainage bag. This way sediment or pus is forced out toward the drainage bag and not toward the bladder.

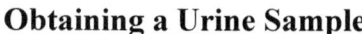

Obtaining a Urine Sample

When the doctor orders a urine specimen for a suspected infection for someone with an indwelling catheter it is necessary to get a sterile specimen. This is done by using the special sampling port found on the side of the catheter. Clamp the tubing below the port, allowing fresh, uncontaminated urine to collect in the tube. After wiping the port with an alcohol pad, insert a sterile syringe hub and withdraw at least 3 to 5 ml. of urine. Using sterile technique, transfer the urine to a sterile container. This could be a sterile specimen cup or a sterile tube.

Never collect a urine specimen from the catheter bag unless it is a brand new sterile bag that has just been taken out of its package and connected to the catheter and you are taking the first urine to go into the bag for your sample.

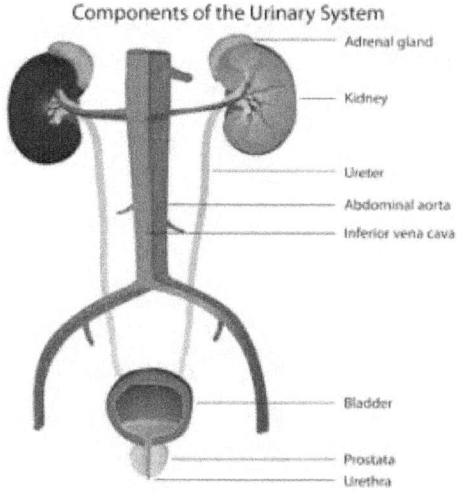

Components of the Urinary System

Adrenal gland

Kidney

Ureter

Abdominal aorta

Inferior vena cava

Bladder

Prostata

Urethra

Preventing Infection

Catheter based infections can be very serious and can even cause death. There are ways to prevent these infections. The number one way is to always wash your hands before and after handling the catheter and/or any part of the drainage system. Remind anyone else who is caring for this person to do the same. Also, wear gloves when indicated and make sure your equipment is cleaned well. Older persons with indwelling catheters may not present with the typical s/s of infection. Very often they will present with mental changes, lethargy, confusion and agitation before any other signs and symptoms.

How do disease causing microorganisms get into the urinary system to cause an Infection? They can get in around the catheter or through the catheter. Getting in around the catheter can happen at the time of insertion or when catheter care is not being done or done properly. Getting in through the catheter usually happens during the time the catheter bag is being emptied. The bag gets on the floor or the connections are not cleansed with alcohol when disconnected.

Some other ways to prevent infections include:

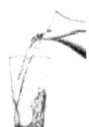

- Drink plenty of fluids: Adults should drink 9 to 13 cups of liquid each day unless restricted by the doctor. One cup is 8 ounces and there is 30 cc or ml in each ounce. Water, juice and milk are the best choices, but coffee, soup and fruit may also count in your daily liquid.
- Keep your drainage system closed. By this I mean do not let any of the connections come apart. Keeping it closed will help to prevent germs from getting into the system.

- Keep your catheter secured by using a catheter strap or tape to secure the catheter to your body. This way the catheter will drain properly.
- Perform catheter care every day or more often if needed i.e. after every bowel movement.

When to Contact the Doctor

- Urgency, frequency, pain, tenderness
- Fever 101 or higher, chills
- Color or changes in the urine such as sediment, pus, blood, bad odor.
- Catheter bag does not fill after several hours.
- Urine leaks around the catheter
- Bladder spasms! These are caused by the balloon irritating the bladder. Signs of these are urge to urinate, leaking urine around the catheter, cramps in the bladder, pain in the penis or vaginal area.
- Catheter comes out.
- There is a layer of crystals inside the tubing.

Removing an indwelling catheter

 An indwelling catheter is removed when the doctor determines that the person should be able to urinate on his or her own. It is also removed when it needs to be changed. This would be 4-12 weeks or when a specific problem dictates it being changed. However, the drainage bag should be changed more frequently – every week? Medicare or insurance might dictate this.

Gather Supplies: 10 ml syringe, disposable gloves, basin of warm water, soap, washcloth and towel

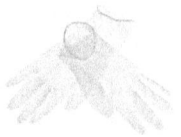

Procedure:

- Put on gloves
- Remove any tape securing the catheter to the patient.
- Attach the syringe to the balloon port on the catheter.
- Slowly withdraw all the contents of the balloon. This deflates the balloon and allows the catheter to be easily removed through the urethra.
- Ask the person to take a deep breath as you gently but firmly pull out the catheter
- Discard gloves, catheter, and drainage bag.
- Provide perineal care.
- Wash hands.

Suprapubic Catheters

A Suprapubic catheter is another type of indwelling catheter. It is a catheter, (sterile tube) that is surgically placed through an opening (stoma) in the abdominal wall. It drains urine out of the bladder into a urinary drainage bag which is attached to the catheter. It is held in place in the bladder by a small balloon that is filled with solution. This system is also a closed drainage system when there are no leaks or disconnections. This system will prevent germs from getting into the urinary system. Keep the catheter tube secured to the body and below the level of the waist so it will drain well. Empty the drainage bag as needed. Do not let it get too full. The weight of a full drainage bag can pull on the stoma and cause injury.

Cleaning the Stoma

Gather supplies: warm water and soap, clean washcloth, clean towel, new gauze pad for dressing if used, disposable gloves

Procedure:

- Wash hands and put on gloves
- Gently remove old dressing around the stoma if there is one.
- Look for redness, drainage, or any skin issues.
- Throw old dressing and gloves in trash.
- Wash hands and put on clean gloves
- Hold the end of the catheter tube at the stoma site so that it doesn't get pulled out while the skin is being cleaned.
- Clean the skin around the stoma using a circular motion moving away from the insertion site.
- Rinse and pat dry and apply bandage if indicated.
- Clean the catheter tube by starting at the insertion site and moving away from the site. Only go in the one direction, away from the site. Do not wash toward the insertion site. This brings the germs back to where you started.
- Secure catheter with tape or catheter strap to leg or abdomen. Do not kink or block the tubing

Problems That Might Occur with a Suprapubic Catheter

- Catheter comes out accidentally: If this happens, a new catheter must be put in right away because the stoma will start to close after about 10 minutes without a catheter in it. Always keep an extra catheter handy.
- The catheter or tubing is blocked: keep the tubing in a straight line when hanging the catheter bag, increase fluid intake, change position of drainage bag
- Urine leaking from stoma or urethra: this may be a sign of infection if a lot of urine is leaking so notify nurse or doctor.
- No urine draining from the catheter: Check the tubing for kinks and make sure the urine bag and tubing are placed below the level of the waist, change body position.

Call nurse or doctor for following

- You have a fever 101 or higher.
- Urine looks or smells bad or has blood in it.
- Changes in mental status.
- The insertion site is red, has a discharge, has an odor, or is bleeding.
- Pain in hip, back, pelvic area, or lower abdomen.

Conclusion

Now that I have taken you through how to care for someone with an indwelling urinary catheter, I hope that you will feel comfortable giving care to someone who has a catheter. This is a common intervention in the home, but it does have its risks. We have discussed the risks and how to prevent them. What I can't stress enough is proper handwashing before and after touching the catheter.

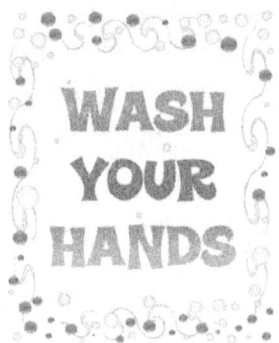

Good Luck!

Resources

www.cdc.gov

www.apic.org

www.caregiver.com

www.caringinfo.org/caringforsomeone

National kidney Foundation - www.kidney.org

About the author

Sharon Kelly is a Registered Nurse who is currently working with nursing students at a local Community College. She has done hospital nursing, home health & hospice nursing, and nursing education. She may be contacted at:

www.skillsfornurses.com

www.thehomecarer.com

www.ingramcontent.com/pod-product-compliance
Lightning Source LLC
Chambersburg PA
CBHW051423170526
45165CB00004BA/1940